divine DIALOGUES

Insights from the Edge

WHAT BEING NEAR DEATH
CAN TEACH US!

SUE PIGHINI

Copyright © 2024 by SUE PIGHINI
All rights reserved.

No part of this book may be reproduced or transmitted in any form or by any means, electronic or mechanical, including photocopying, recording, or by any information storage and retrieval system, without permission in writing from the copyright owner.

Table of Contents

Preface *vii*
Maryanne Williamson Quote *xi*
Introduction *xiii*

Part I
The Stories from the Edge

Chapter 1 Story #1: Lightning in Arizona *3*

Chapter 2 Story #2: Guns in New York City *7*

Chapter 3 Story #3: Near Death in Virginia *13*

Part II
Bella and her Angelic Friends' Blogs

Chapter 1 What is Your Vibration *21*

Chapter 2 There Are Two of You *25*

Chapter 3 Your Wings Are Ready *29*

Chapter 4 Your Soul Speaks *31*

Chapter 5 What Your Life Demands *35*

Chapter 6 Being Human is No Cakewalk *39*

Chapter 7 We Are Becoming a "DIY" Society *43*

Chapter 8 Creating Greater Personal Freedom *47*

Chapter 9 Your God Connection *51*

Part III
Dancing with the Divine

In Gratitude   *61*

Images   *63*

DIVINE DIALOGUES

You Are Never Alone!
YOU are the creator and designer of your life and ALL that is in it!

Live well! Design well!

Love yourself – YOU are EXTRAORDINARY!
With extraordinary gifts and talents to share with the world!

"*Nothing great in this world has ever been accomplished without Passion.*"
Hebel – poet

Divine Dialogues
Preface

I started writing this book in 2020 when we were just beginning to see the extraordinary challenges of COVID-19. I wanted to share the wisdom of what I call the Angelic Realm messages. So, I decided to tackle a third book, "Divine Dialogues". Since 1972, with a lightning strike literally under my belt, I have been receiving guidance from some unknown source about how to live my life with greater courage and take more chances for change. From 1972 to 2016, I have had 3 near-death experiences and several STEs (spiritually transformative experiences). Thus, the downloaded guidance that I write and speak about.

One of the key gifts of this Angelic wisdom happened in 2000 when I was living on an island and wanted to find something new to do in my life (I had just retired from corporate life). So, I volunteered to help a friend groom and walk horses. I knew nothing about horses. But that June day in 2000, my life changed forever and has been changing every day since.

My friend said, "Go into the barn and look at the horses in the stalls and decide which one you would like to groom (which I knew nothing about). I will then teach you how to touch them (really?) and gain their trust." I did what she said. I walked into this lovely barn and walked over to the stalls, and immediately, I connected with a very large black horse who stuck his head out and seemed to say, "Pick me! Pick me!" So, I did!

One of the best experiences of my life! The smell of his coat, his gorgeous deep black eyes, and his sweet muzzle (nose) were more than I could handle. I started to tear up! Why? That day in June was the beginning of life as a horsewoman – at age 60! I have been loving and working with horses ever since. It is never too late to find your passion in life. And, this step into the equine world is, to this day, a step into the divine nature of our world. And a deep passion for me.

I am telling you this because I just learned in March 2023, that my passion for these extraordinary animals has led me again to believe in miracles. When I survived the lightning strike in 1972, being held up at gunpoint in 1984, and a brain aneurysm in 2016, I felt that each of these events was a miracle in itself. All are recounted in Part I of this book.

In 2020, we had to sell our farm in Virginia due to my husband's poor health and move to Florida, which we both love. Our 5 beautiful horses were donated to a wonderful, loving nonprofit in Pennsylvania. Every single day, I would wake up with tears in my eyes and the vision of each horse in my mind. I loved them so much. I missed them so much. It just didn't make any sense that we could have kept them. It was just so much work and expense, but I loved them so much.

It was now March 2023 and I got a text on a Sunday from the Pennsylvania nonprofit that they sadly must find a new home for the horses. COVID had forced them to close their doors. My husband and I were stunned, but we both said, in unison, "No new home for them. They are coming back to us in Florida." We had to find a place to board them, someone to trailer them down here and figure out how we would pay for their future. We are retired! Within one week, we found a boarding farm to bring them to and a wonderful and safe equine transport company to bring them here to us, and we would have to dip into our savings to find the money.

Preface

We are in our mid-70's and this is an absolute miracle to have them back with us. We both are thrilled and I can't believe how much more energy we have just being in their presence.

The wisdom of this story is that LOVE is the strongest energy in the universe. When you love something so much that you will do whatever it takes to manifest that "thing," it will happen. Warren Buffet – money. Lady Gaga – to be able to sing in any venue, any time. Stephen Hawking – to discover the Black Hole in space regardless of his deteriorating physical condition.

YOU ARE EXTRAORDINARY! Love your life! Discover the things in life that give you freedom, happiness and joy. Life is about Passion and Purpose! The stronger those feelings are, the faster they will manifest into the physical.

This book is about how I was shown to connect with the Angelic Realm through my NDE experiences and through the wisdom and energy of horses—as I call them, our Fabulous Five! My passion in this lifetime is all about partnering with these horses to help bring YOU and others the guidance to maximize your gifts and talents by finding your unique path to peace and joy. Every day that I am with them, I receive messages on how to share their divine wisdom with you.

In Part II, I have compiled these wonderful Angelic messages from 2020–2023, which have been energetically enhanced and edited by being with the horses again, especially Ms. Bella, our youngest. Bella's energy of love for the human and her innate wisdom has enhanced my ability to receive these Angelic insights.

I hope you enjoy this journey through the wisdom of the horse and the Angelic Realm as much as I do and that it resonates with you in an extraordinary way.

Our Deepest Fear

Our deepest fear is not that we are inadequate. Our deepest fear is that we are powerful beyond measure. It is our light, not our darkness, that most frightens us. We ask ourselves, who am I to be brilliant, gorgeous, talented, and fabulous? Actually, who are you not to be? You are a child of God. Your playing small does not serve the world. There is nothing enlightened about shrinking so that other people won't feel insecure around you. We are all meant to shine, as children do. We were born to make manifest the glory of God that is within us. It is not just in some of us; it is in everyone. And as we let our own light shine, we unconsciously give other people permission to do the same. As we are liberated from our own fear, our presence automatically liberates others.

— *Marianne Williamson*

"Divine Dialogues"
Introduction
My Story and How It Might Resonate with You!

From The Angelic Realm: "You are Extraordinary!"
I certainly didn't know what "extraordinary" meant in 1972 when I was suddenly struck by lightning in the Arizona mountains. I was an incredibly young and naïve wife and mother, 27 years old, in a very dysfunctional marriage. My life was a mess and was totally changed in a split second. I was saved by an ancient-sounding voice, which I call Angelic, that told me to move my legs back and forth, back and forth across the mud, to save my heart from the "fire" of the lightning coursing through my body. *I was having a near-death experience.* I had no idea what that meant either. I had never heard of near death before. I just knew I had touched the "other side." This exceptional event put me on a path of searching for the meaning of my life. Why was I still alive? Why was I here? Just like you, I wanted to know if heaven was real, if angels were real. Little did I know that this experience was just the beginning of having my questions answered.

Then, in 2016, after launching my second book, "Expect the Extraordinary," I was on a radio interview and saw a huge ball of white lightning come across the pasture and enter my forehead. What *was* that? Whatever it was, I was on the floor, having trouble breathing. I found my cell phone next to me and speed-dialed my husband. With his medical background, he knew immediately that I was having a brain aneurysm. It was nine days in intensive care before the neurosurgeon could find the bleed in a very obscure location behind my right ear. As I was going into the third exploratory surgery, I was just *so* tired. I just wanted to rest – forever. Too much, too overwhelming. As I was getting prepped for the final angiogram procedure, there appeared 12 small, childlike Angelic beings, all smiling in a white glow, around the surgical table. And, one very large being in white to my right over my shoulder. "We have you. You are safe. You are loved." With a huge smile on his face. The love was palpable and electric. *I was having my second near-death experience.*

It was now 2019 and I had just found out that I had skin cancer for the second time. On my nose and it had to be removed immediately. (I had put it off, being human and all.) This was a two-part surgery, three weeks apart. Part one was a success as the plastic surgeon removed the basal cell cancer growth without my losing my entire right nostril. Part two was reconstruction. I was really scared before I went into the second surgery, and I couldn't figure out why. It was a quick reconstruction – an hour. But, during recovery, I felt myself slipping away to my right when, all of a sudden, I was shaking violently – inside. I struggled to come out of the anesthesia, and when I could finally talk, I asked the nurse what had happened, and she said all went well, no problems. "I was shaking?" *She said no. I was quiet as a mouse.* I then asked to speak to the anesthesiologist, and he came down to recovery. *But, he said, no shaking – quiet as a mouse.* Then, I remembered there were several people at the end of my bed, all dressed in white and a beautiful woman gently holding onto my legs. But – the recovery room staff were all dressed in blue. Who were these people? What happened? *I was having my third near-death experience.* These were Angelic presences - again.

Introduction

But why? Was I trying to slip away again, like in 2016? Why didn't I want to stay?

It is now February 15, 2023, and I am finally getting some clarity on what I am supposed to do with these extraordinary connections. *I am to share them with you.* I didn't slip away because my soul wanted me to stay and finally do the job I chose to do when I was born. To tell everyone I could that: Heaven is REAL. Angels are REAL. They want you to know that they are here for *you* every moment of every day. They want my experiences to help others see that there is another world outside of the massive earthly changes that are taking place globally with COVID-19, race issues, earth changes and political and economic turmoil. They are asking me to share what I have learned over 40 years so that you can connect with the all-loving, all-supportive nonphysical domain of our world. So, let's take a glimpse into the world of the Angelic Realm. Here are some of the "Divine Dialogues" I have been graciously given over the last few years, and even now, every day:

- YOU ARE EXTRAORDINARY! Your soul *chose* to be here on earth at this time to help bring enormous change to our world.

- The catalyst for this change is – LOVE!

- All beings are sacred – animals, human beings, Mother Nature – even your plants and minerals. Love them all!

- Your life is a gift of TODAY, not regrets of yesterday or worries of tomorrow. Breathe life NOW, live life NOW, love life NOW!

- How important is your anger? If you could never hug or talk to that other person that you are angry with, would you still be angry at them? Once you have crossed to the other side, there is no going back. There are no hugs, no touching, no physical loving.

- Simplify, simplify. What are your true necessities in this world? How much "stuff" do you need? Maybe the less fortunate could use your "stuff" to stay warm or dressed. We are all energetically connected, whether from Utah or Uganda.

- Be STILL sometime during your day for 10 minutes. Find gratitude in your heart for all in your life that gives you joy. Forget the challenges. They are learning cycles. Concentrate on the people, animals and events that give you joy. Hug a human, hug a horse!

These messages above are just a few of what I have received over the last many years and, more importantly, in the last three years. I have more Angelic insights in my blogs on my website: www.SuePighini.com and https://bloggingwithsue.com.

Why did I have three near-death experiences? Because I volunteered to be a Messenger of the Heart. Welcoming change and inviting personal growth is my passion and purpose for being here. Every one of us is driven to find our deepest desire, discover who we are, discover our life's mission, and share it with others. Our passion connects us to our Source.

I send each of you love and light during this extraordinary time of challenge and change. Namaste' – the Divine in me honors the Divine in you.

part one

STORIES FROM THE EDGE

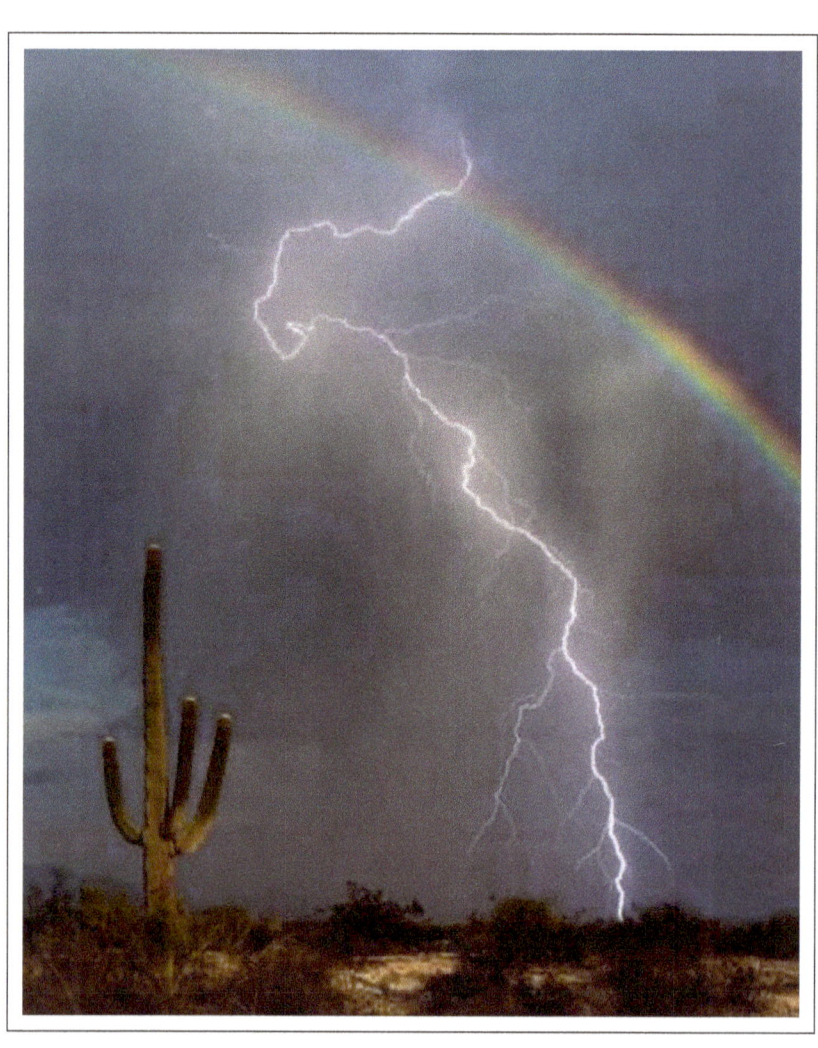

Story #1

"Let There Be Light" in the Arizona Mountains

It's 1972 and I am stuck out in a small Arizona desert town with a Sears Catalogue order showroom. That's how small it was. My military husband, Pete, was stationed at Ft. Huachuca, AZ, training Army troops for overseas deployment. I was stuck in a small house with two darling young children and a disintegrating marriage. How was I going to get out of this suffocating situation? I prayed for help. I begged for guidance. There was nowhere to turn. So, I just had to ride this misery out until I could find some peace somewhere, somehow.

It's now August in Sierra Vista, AZ and we are in the rainy season. My husband was a Special Forces officer and loved to take chances. So, that particular day in August, we were going for a motorcycle ride into the small mountains nearby to look at the Indian caves, even though a major rainstorm was forecasted. These caves were renowned in southern Arizona. We reached the bottom of the cave hill and climbed on our hands and knees to the opening of the grotto and were astounded by the colorful drawings on the walls. How had these beautiful renderings lasted so long? We weren't there 5 minutes when thunder clapped us out of our reverie. My husband yelled that he had to get down the hill to start the bike before it was flooded. He told me to come down as soon as I could, even scooting on my bottom if I had to. I ran outside the cave to find rain coming down in torrents, so powerful that I couldn't see where the bike was. I fell down in the mud and started to scooch down on my rear end. I kept slipping in the mud, so I decided to stand up and grab a nearby fence pole. Lightning struck through the pole, into my right arm and across my body into the ground!

"You can't leave now. You must go back to the children. Move your legs back and forth, back and forth, so the 'fire' doesn't reach your heart." I had to be unconscious. Where am I? I want to go to that bright light right over there, over my right shoulder. I don't want to go back. I feel safe here near the light. But I must go back for Cathy and Chris. My babies! Then, I could feel my legs swinging back and forth in the mud. I could feel the mud in my nose and mouth. And I was so cold. Where were my clothes? The rain was so cold. Where were my clothes?

My husband saw me from the bottom of the hill. He realized what had happened because my clothes were melting off my body and I was steaming. He left the bike running and climbed up to get me, throwing me on his back and holding onto my arms. (I couldn't feel anything at that point).

As the Universe would have it, there was a logging cabin near the mountain that we had seen coming up. Pete rushed the bike there and parked, carrying me inside to get out of the freezing rain. He found firewood stacked in a corner but no way to light it. Just then, we heard more motorcycles outside the cabin door. Two men raced inside, soaking wet and stared at me with their mouths open – partly because I had very few clothes still on my body. They had disintegrated on the ride down the mountain. Pete told them what had happened and they found a metal bucket in a corner and hurried back outside to empty gas from their cycles. A fire was finally started and I could feel some warmth finally. My teeth had stopped chattering, but my body was still shaking. The guys brought in some dry clothes for me from their saddle bags, and oh, they felt so good and dry. In the meantime, my husband called 911 from the cabin phone for an ambulance to come up the hill to get me. Because of the relentless rain, they said getting up the hill would be close to impossible. But they would try their absolute best. About an hour later, we could hear the ambulance labor up the hill to the fire cabin. They came running inside, took my vital signs, put me on a gurney and whisked me away to the hospital at Ft. Huachuca. As the doctors examined me, they kept telling me how lucky I was. Why? I asked. "Because we lost two young climbers last month in the exact same location from lightning strikes. You are one incredibly lucky woman." And, so the miracles began.

Madison Av

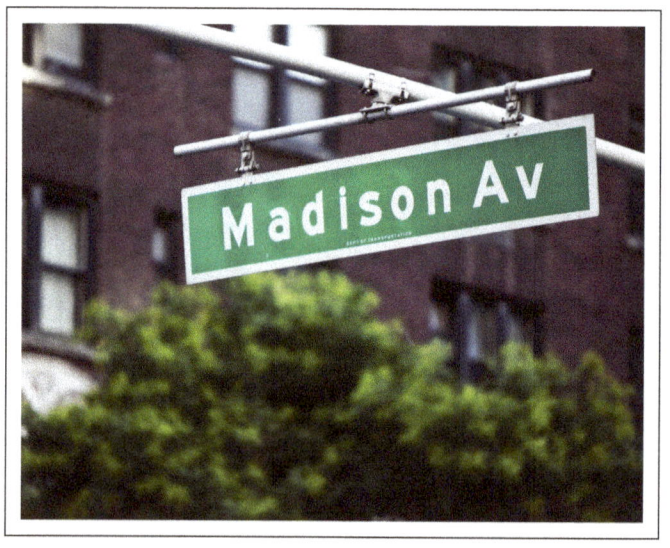

Story #2

Guns on Madison Avenue, New York City

This particular story is about a spiritually transformative experience (STE) vs an NDE. An STE is an event where you encounter a spiritual entity or vision but do not always travel to or connect with the light of the non-physical world. I have had several STE's, but this special one in New York City saved my life.

What a beautiful night in New York City! It was warm and in the low 70s in early October! I was enormously happy. I had a great new job and an even better new relationship. After the lightning accident several years earlier, I stayed in my marriage to Pete for six more years, knowing that it wasn't working and that I was too afraid to leave. When I finally decided that I could raise Cathy and Chris on my own, the floodgates of employment opportunities just opened up for me (starting with selling tennis racquets and jock straps. Wow! What a thrilling opportunity!). Peter and I divorced. I held several jobs in New York City before I finally found my dream job with a marketing company based in New York and Connecticut and literally headquartered down the street from where I lived in Westport, CT. Amazing, synchronicity at its finest!

My new relationship was with Bob Kipperman, and it would turn into an engagement and a 28-year marriage before he passed away in 2007 from a rare heart disease. But this particular night in

New York was magical. We had eaten at a great Italian restaurant, Il Menestrello, and were just strolling up Madison Avenue to the apartment of a friend on Madison and 83rd. The friend graciously offered up his one-bedroom condo for us to stay in for the weekend. We both had been working so hard and then commuting every night home on the train back to Connecticut. Bob worked as a vice president at CBS Television, so he was always in a stressful situation. The weekend getaway was such a treat, just what we needed.

As we strolled up Madison from 50th Street, it would take us about an hour to slowly make our way to 83rd Street. We were kibitzing about my new job and Bob's upcoming trip to a televised golf tournament. We were holding hands, with each of our briefcases being carried by our outside hands, as we reached 80th and Madison. Suddenly, a tall, skinny man and a short, extremely nervous younger man came up behind us and said, "Back up against the fence and don't do anything stupid, like try to get attention from the people walking across the street." I was dumbfounded. What was happening? Were these jokers real, and were they robbing us on Madison Avenue? The next sentence confirmed it. Tall Guy said, "Give me all your jewelry and your money. Where's your wallet, Mr. Big Shot? Give it to me." Bob was in shock, too, because he said, "Don't take her jewelry; it was a gift." The Tall One just howled with laughter. "OK, I'll send it to my mama for safekeeping." Short Guy was just standing next to Tall Guy, holding the gun, with his arm shaking like a leaf. This must have been his initiation into the world of big-time crime. I started to take off my new necklace (a recent gift from Bob) when Tall Guy just reached over and yanked it off my neck. That yank really hurt—the necklace had a thick gold chain on it. I could feel the panic rising up inside of me. These guys were serious!

Suddenly, a voice broke through my terror. In my head, I could hear: "Fall to the ground on your knees. Tell them you are pregnant, and you are going to vomit and be sick all over the sidewalk. Do it now!" The voice was gentle but very urgent. It wasn't the same voice that came to me when I was struck by lightning. It was firmer, stronger. I did exactly as I was told. I fell to the sidewalk and yelled, "I am pregnant. I'm going to be sick." Bob almost had a heart attack and said, "Sue, not now!" (He knew I wasn't pregnant.) Tall Guy said, "Get up, Lady, now, or I will blow your head off." I answered, "I can't. I am so sick. You'll have to shoot me." He was so startled by what I said that he looked around and could see people on the other side of Madison Avenue stopping and staring at us. He finally said, "I don't know if you're really sick, Lady, but we got everything we came for. We are outta here." Saving face! So important! Then, they slowly sauntered off laughing across Madison to Fifth Avenue and The Metropolitan Museum of Art.

Bob was so jacked up and furious that we had been robbed that he took off his suit jacket, handed it to me and said he was going after them. I couldn't believe it and begged him to call 911 instead. But he took off running and yelled back at me to go to the nearest restaurant and call 911. I ran over to the other side of the street, found a small Greek deli, and asked to use the phone because we had just been robbed. This was before cell phones, of course. I finally connected with 911, and they sent police squad cars racing up the wrong way on Fifth Avenue to the Museum. I ran over to the Museum carrying two briefcases and Bob's jacket while three police cars jumped the sidewalk in front of me and took off down the museum sidewalk. The police piled out of their squad cars and surrounded the suspects, who gave up immediately with six guns pointed at them and more coming. Bob was ushered back to where I was standing and then yelled to the police, "Here's the gun, on the ground by the bushes. Let me have it—I'll kill them." A little adrenaline speaking up! The gun was retrieved, but nowhere could they find the stolen jewelry.

The police pushed the two suspects into two separate squad cars while they looked for the necklace and Bob's wallet. Suddenly, one of the cops yanked Tall Guy out of the squad car and furiously pulled out the back seat. There, sitting under the backseat cushion, were the wallet and the necklace. Now, they had all they needed—stolen items and the gun.

We finally got to our friend's apartment at about midnight. Bob never went to sleep—he was too keyed up. I, on the other hand, had one glass of wine, and I was out until the phone rang at 6am. It was my babysitter in Connecticut telling us that the Manhattan police were looking for us. She gave us the phone number of the precinct who had called, and Bob called them back. They wanted us to come up to the Police Headquarters immediately. Something had come up, and they needed identity confirmation of the thieves right away. A squad car was sent to pick us up with the same detective who had overseen the case from the night before. We felt safer knowing that the same guy who captured these crazies would be there for us. They didn't tell us right away what was happening. When we got to the precinct, they just put each of us in separate rooms to question us. They showed us photos of each guy and asked if we recognized either of them. We both firmly confirmed that they were the two guys who held us up. Then, they told us why we had been brought in. Tall Guy had murdered two Hispanic doormen on the West Side of Manhattan two weeks before because they didn't have enough money on them to make it worth Tall Guy's time. We both were stunned.

We could have died right there on Madison Avenue at 8:30 on a Friday night. That urgent Angelic voice saved us. When Bob asked me later why I dropped to the ground with a gun pointed at my head, I told him about the Whisper. He didn't believe me. I don't know if I believed it, either. But, several years later, when my life was saved again by another voice, I knew someone was trying to give me a message. But what message? What am I supposed to do with these messages? In 1988, I finally realized these communications were given to me to get my attention and to share with others how each of us have Angelic saviors who want to connect with us. They are here to protect and love us – we just have to listen carefully, because sometimes they whisper.

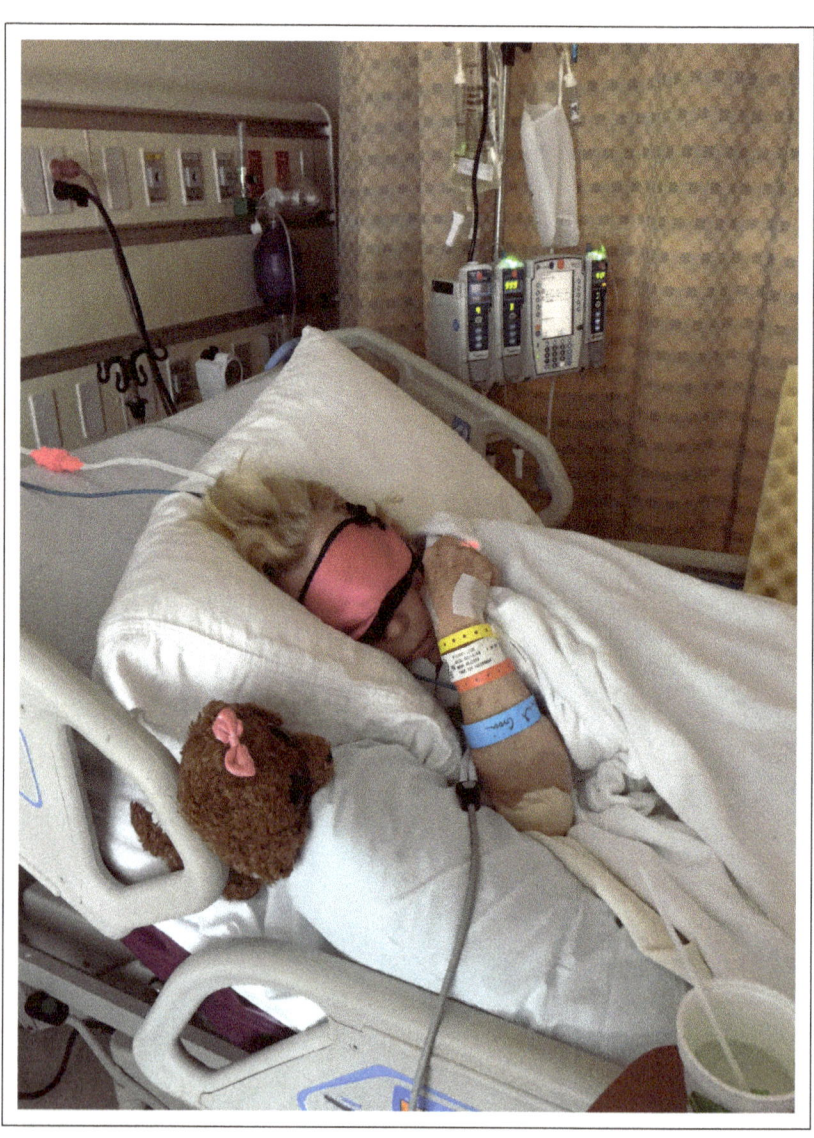

Story #3

Near Death in Virginia

It is now 2016, and I am remarried to John Pighini, decorated Air Force Special Operator, as Bob passed away in 2008 from a rare heart disease that he had been fighting for 10 years. I have just finished publishing "Expect the Extraordinary," a book introducing the reader to near death and what it is all about - loving guidance and help from the non-physical or "the other side," as I call it. I was promoting this second book on the radio, podcasts and zoom calls and was super busy just coming back from New York City at a promotional seminar.

It was a beautiful day in May, the 17th to be exact, and I was on a radio interview on the phone, looking out my office window, watching the horses play in the front pasture. When, all of a sudden, a huge white ball of light races across the pasture, comes through the window and into my forehead. I was stunned. What just happened? Then, I knew I really didn't feel well. I told the radio host interviewing me that I might have the stomach flu and had to hang up. Just laid the phone down on the floor, I fell down, unconscious. I came to shortly after, pulled my phone over to me and speed dialed John. We had help at the farm and John called Rachel and she came running in. I couldn't really speak much but she told me John had called 911 and told them he thought I had a brain aneurysm. He had a medical background from the military as a retired Air Force Pararescueman.

Shortly after, 911 came running in, cut my clothes off and started running tests. I felt so sick. I just couldn't stop vomiting. They whisked me off on a gurney and on the way to the local Fredericksburg, Virginia hospital. John was already there to meet me and asked the attending/visiting neurosurgeon from Walter Reed what he would do if it was his wife. He said that Walter Reed didn't have the absolute best diagnostic equipment for aneurysms of the brain. He would call his friend, Dr. Dennis Rivet, head of neurosurgery at Virginia Commonwealth Hospital in Richmond, VA, to see if they could take me right now. Their equipment was top-notch and the absolute newest in the industry. The neurosurgeon called, and VCU *could* admit me, and we were on our way, by ambulance vs. chopper because of severe weather. I don't remember too much of the hospital until the next day when I tried to get up and walk out – with the IV pole still attached to my arm. Boy – didn't the bells go off then? Nurses were everywhere. They cleaned up the blood and got me back in bed, and, most probably, medicated me thoroughly to keep me still.

I met Dr. Rivet the next day, and he then performed a cerebral angiogram searching for the brain bleed. No luck! Couldn't find it. We are now on day five, and no good news. Day 7, another angiogram is performed. Still, no luck. Dr. Rivet comes in and says, "We can't find that small vessel that is giving us the problem. I have spent two days researching this type of aneurysm, and you, My Dear, are one of 15 people in the last 25 years who have survived this event. Would you trust me to go back in one more time? I think I know where it might be."

Me: "Do I have a choice? Please do the best that you can—I have a lot of people and animals depending on me. I trust you."

We are now on day 9 in ICU. I am getting prepped each day for the surgery, but there are numerous delays. Other emergency patients are coming in hourly. With no food and very little water for

Story #3: Near Death in Virginia

two days, I say to John: "I don't think I can do this anymore. I am so tired." He says: "Don't you dare leave me!"

I am finally being prepped in the OR for the third time after 9 days, and being transferred to the operating table. Suddenly, I see 12 small Angels in glowing white surrounding the table. They are all smiling and looking at me, as if there is nothing to be worried about. Then, standing above and next to my right shoulder is an exceptionally large Angelic being in white who I know is familiar. He says, "We have you, and you are loved." It is Jesus. I think I have seen him many times before, in meditative dreams.

The surgery was a success. The brain bleed was from an exceedingly small vessel behind my right ear. Three titanium coils were inserted, and now, eight years later, I have an extraordinary life. It took more than a year to feel normal from all of the meds and surgeries, and my riding my horses has been severely curtailed. But I am alive and living my life exploring every new excitement I can find. I teach a course entitled "Light Your Life on Fire." It talks about taking chances to find your Passion and Purpose in life, and finding gratitude in each day, even if it's a challenging day like living through Covid and its aftermath.

The Angelic presence is with me daily. I sometimes think I can hear their laughter at my worries. They say, "It's all about learning and wisdom—there's no need to worry".

I feel strongly that I must share these stories with you, my reader, because I don't want you to be afraid of death. It is so peaceful if we ask for "ease and grace" during our transition. You don't have to be struck by lightning, be held up at gunpoint or suffer a brain aneurysm to touch the amazing nonphysical world that deeply loves us and lifts us up in our most challenging times. *You are a child of God and are here to light up the world with your gifts and talents. Know how especially important you are to this world.*

With deep love to each of you. . . . . . Sue

part two

BLOGS FROM SWEET BELLA AND HER ANGELIC FRIENDS

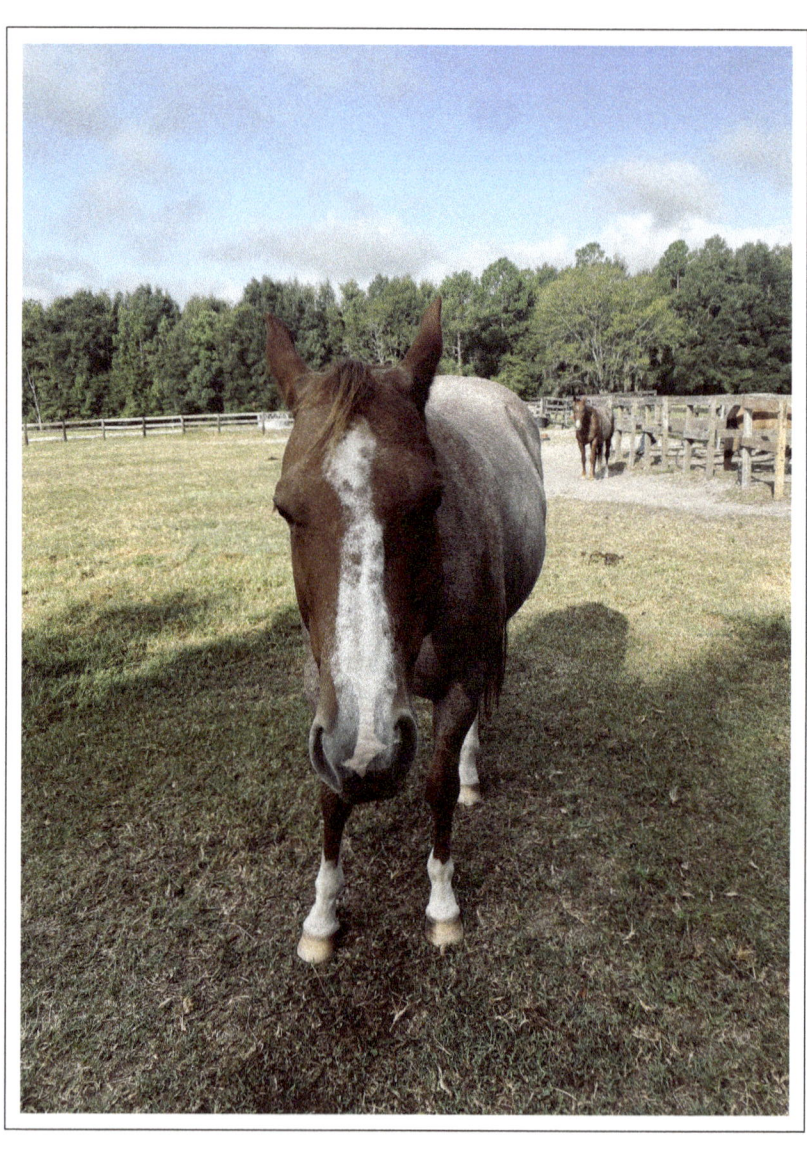

COVID Blogs from Sweet Bella and her Angelic Friends

2019–2022

During COVID-19, when we were all housebound and couldn't go to our normal places of work or activities, I began spending more time with our horses, The Fabulous Five. I particularly concentrated on Bella, our youngest, who was 6 at the time. After a few months, I realized that I kept getting impulses to write down what I call messages from the nonphysical when I was spending time with her. Thus, Sue's Blogs were born. Bella's young energy of pure love, along with my NDE experiences, opened my energy system to receive "downloads" from the universe.

What I have compiled from the many messages I received are the 9 that I thought you might find thought provoking. I hope you enjoy them and find them helpful in your pursuit of personal freedom and spiritual expansion.

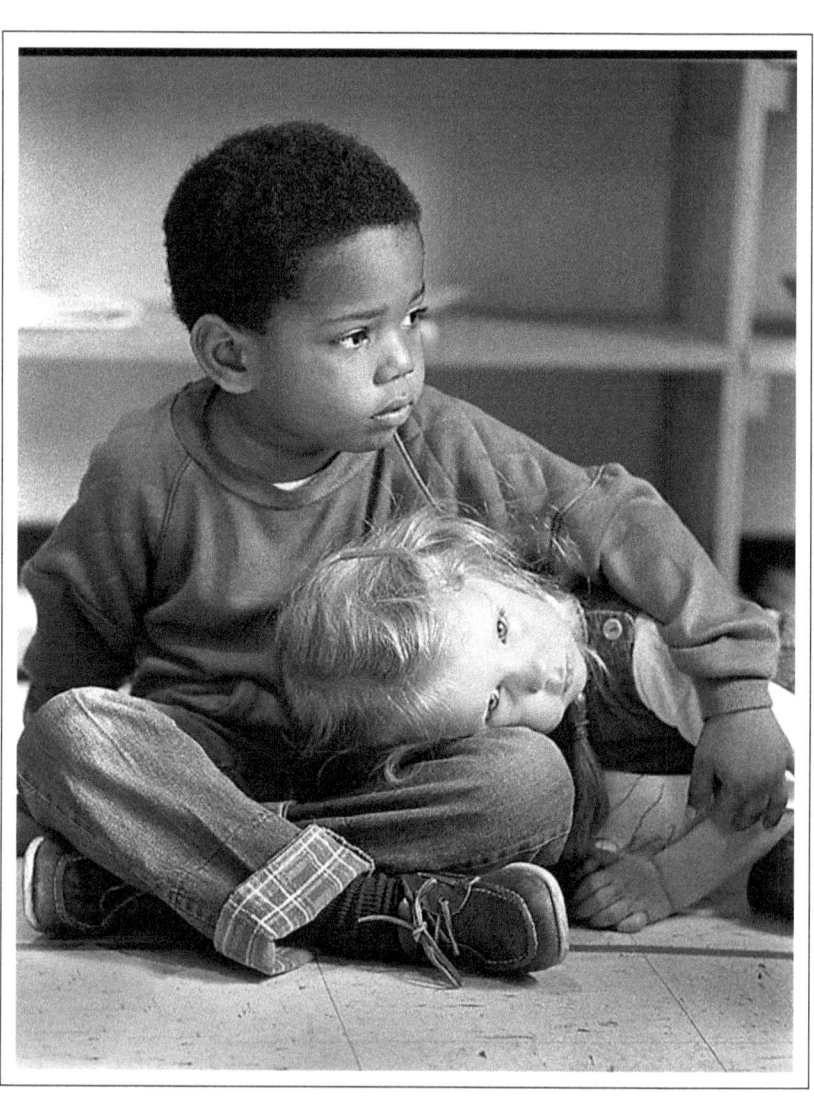

Blog #1

What Is Your Vibration in this Extraordinary Time?

What is *your* personal vibration? Why is it important? The attached image touches our hearts with the vibration of love, regardless of the color of our skin, our religious preferences or the language we speak. Your vibration is your "calling card" or essence of who you are. It is your thought patterns mixed in with your desires for the future. It is like a radio tower putting out radio signals of who you are and why you are here.

Not only do we have COVID-19 to challenge us, but our understanding of loving ALL of humanity and all beings has come into global vibration with the unbelievably sad passing of George Floyd. What an enormous sacrifice he has made to bring us to this point of understanding that there is NO separation from each other regardless of beliefs, language or skin color. We are all children of God from the same Source.

The Angels speak now:

- YOU are extraordinary!
- You are a vessel of love. THAT WAS YOUR VIBRATION AT BIRTH!

- The vibration of your love can transform the lives of others. A simple smile is all it takes.

- When you honor *your life,* you honor *all lives.*

- Your honoring of life can change the vibration of the earth and the safety and peace of its inhabitants.

- Every day, do something that gives you GREAT JOY!

- Do not go back to the past to find happiness. It is in today.

- TODAY is the day to build your vibration to a higher level of inclusiveness. Love ALL! Honor ALL!

- Tomorrow is what dreams are made of. WHAT IS YOUR LIFETIME DREAM? Act on every dream that gives you an uplifting, passionate feeling coming from your heart. This is your original vibration: LOVE!

And you ask "What if I fall?"
Oh but my darling,
What if you fly?
Erin Hanson
horse tricks 101

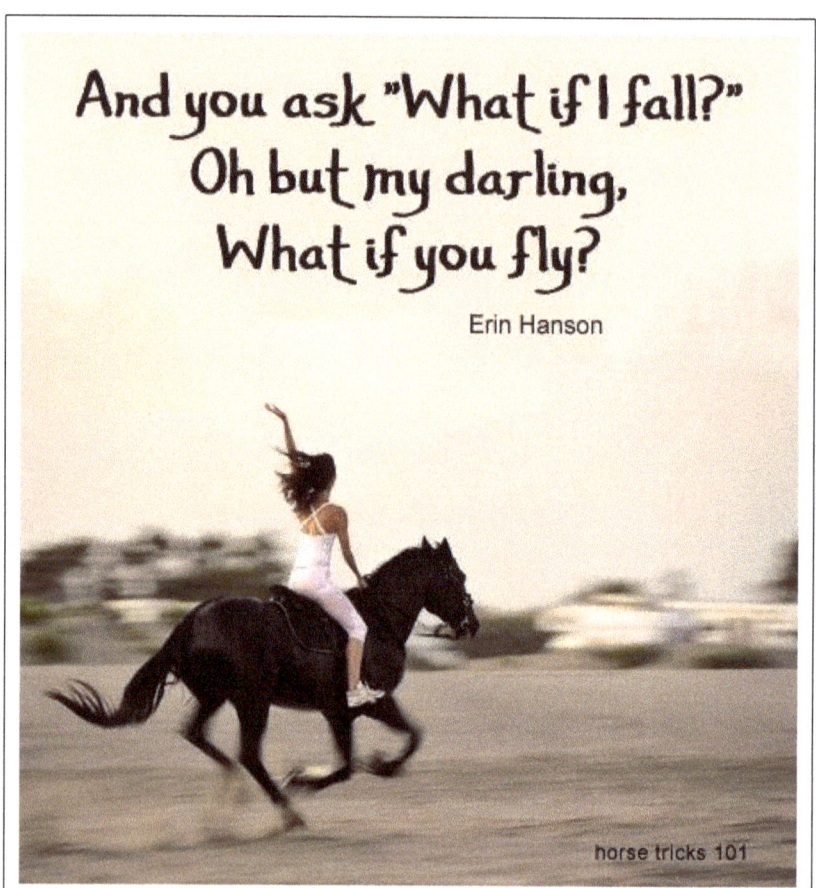

Blog #2

2019: There Are Two of YOU! Who Are They?

There are two of you—your physical self and your spiritual self. During this time of challenge, the Angels want to communicate with you about which self will help you most deal with the daily changes. Your spiritual self is the part of you that will come forward when you operate from your heart and your intuition, not ever from fear. Making the best decisions for you and your family comes from a place of compassion for your environment and what's happening and *from the honoring of all other beings.*

From the Angels:

- "YOU ARE EXTRAORDINARY!
- When you offer compassion or honor to others regardless of who they are or what they look like, you are operating from your *spiritual self.*
- Remember that all beings, human or animal, have information or learning for you.
- BUT—before you can honor others, you must honor yourself. Our non-physical realm loves you beyond measure. We are ALWAYS with you.

- What is your passion in life? What excites you? That passion will help heal you and others around you. Act on your drive to be all you can be! Now, as we pause in our society, ask yourself what REALLY matters to you. Are you doing what YOU LOVE?

- YOU are extraordinary! Be safe, be well and know that you are loved beyond measure!"

From Sue:

- *For more than 40 years, the Angelic Realms have coached and coerced me to voice their wisdom. COVID-19 has propelled me to do just that. I hope these messages bring you comfort and the realization that you are so much more than you know. Enjoy these recent changes as our world is spun into new adventures of light and love. Change is always a bit challenging!*

YOUR TIME AS A CATERPILLAR IS OVER
YOUR WINGS AWAIT

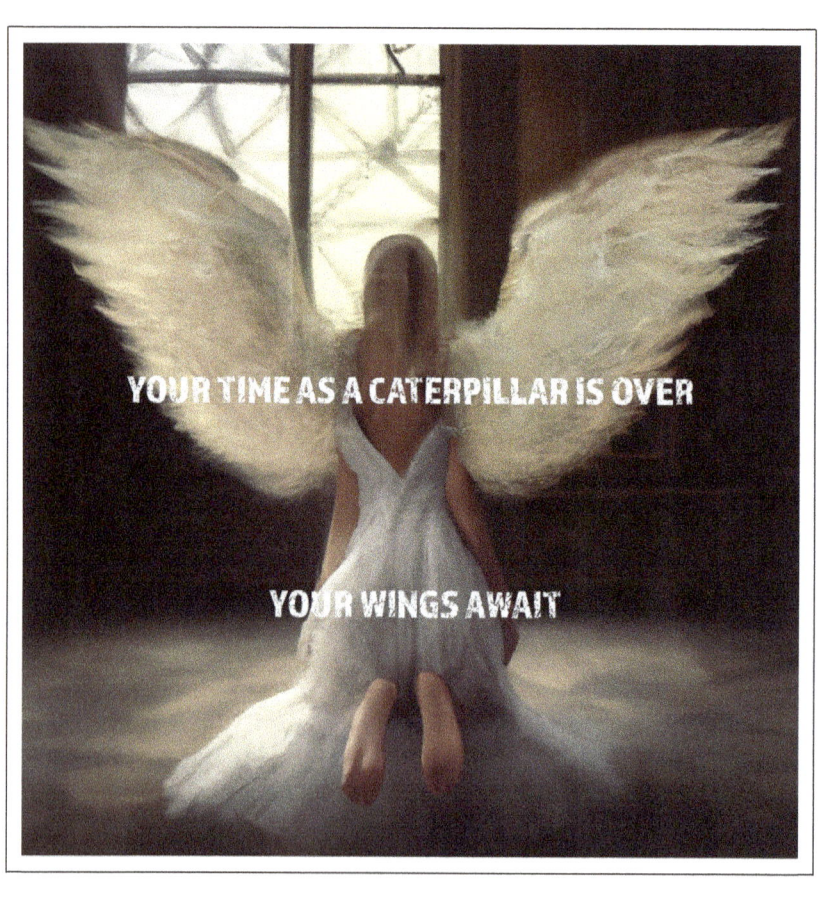

Blog #3

Your Wings Are Ready!

"YOU ARE EXTRAORDINARY! You are a light in the darkness and a breath of fresh air in the suffocating chaos of world changes that are taking place. For you to be all you want to be, it is time to take new chances and live more fearlessly. Are you happy where you live? With whom you live? What your job/work might be? All of these things are indicators of how you live in happiness. Each of these things can be heightened and made more fulfilling with conversation/connection with others. You are energetically, invisibly aligned with everyone, everywhere and they teach you, and you teach them. What are you learning from them? From the news? From life around you?

   As you desire to make changes in your life, can nature help you live more intuitively? Talk to your dog, your cat, your horse, your flowers. They all have energy there to help you become all you desire to be. It is the natural ORDER of things. It is divine vibration. Feel the intuitive hits you receive and write them down. This is not about perfection but about being all you can be. You are a divine human angel being loved by all other divine beings, physical and non-physical!"

BE safe, be well!
With love and light,
Sue

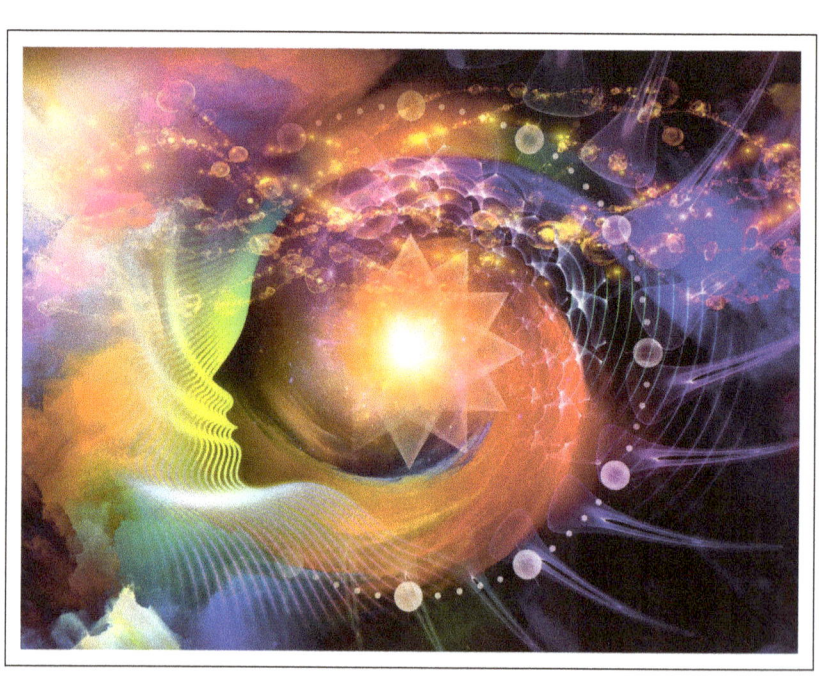

Blog #4

Your Soul Speaks!

The Angels speak:
"The attached image is one of *your soul* looking down on you in human form from its home in the non-physical Universe. 90% of your soul is in the non-physical and 10% is here on earth. The 90% soul is constantly learning from its 10% self as you go through your life. So, the question becomes: Why are you here? What did you come to learn for your soul's growth? Here is a KEY:

You and your soul CHOSE to be here during this time of unprecedented turmoil: COVID-19, racial unrest, natural earth disasters and economic and political chaos. Why? Because you signed a contract with the Angelic realm and all the millions of souls in the nonphysical realm to come to help initiate enormous change for humanity. These millions of souls put YOU before them because they felt you could do a better job at helping to re-seed love on our planet than they could. WHY? You promised to do whatever it took to rebirth the loving energy of Mother Earth."

From Sue: Now, how do you do this? You learn ALL you can about yourself and your gifts - to share with others.

- <u>*What are your passions?*</u> *How do they make a difference? How can YOU help humanity by sharing your gifts and talents?*

- *You live from your heart in LOVE. <u>I am you and you are me.</u> You and I came from the exact same Source and that same energy runs through all of our veins. See the rioters, the racial dividers, the angry faces as lost to their own hearts. BE ALL YOU CAN BE and your energy will pass along to everyone you meet."*

Be safe. Be well. Know that you are EXTRAORDINARY and loved beyond measure.

If your life demands
that you walk through
hell
walk like you
own the damn place

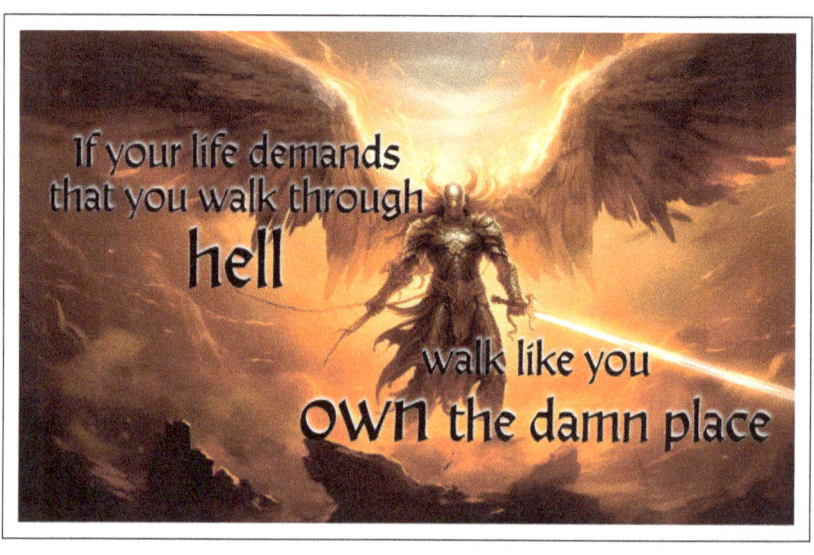

Blog #5

What Your Life Demands!

"If Your *Life* Demands You Walk Through Hell, Walk Like You Own the Damn Place!"

You are extraordinary! These past 2+ years have truly been a physical, emotional, and spiritual challenge/test for us all. But why, at this time, is there so much upheaval? Weather, politics, economies, health challenges with Covid and without - all challenge us to be all we can be. It is tough being human! The Angels applaud us for taking this on, for being here at this time to see how we can make a difference in our own lives and those around us.

From a spiritual perspective, we signed on for this lifetime long before we were born. It is a soul passage that your soul wants to be part of - being alive during this time on earth. It wants to learn and make a difference in its earthly incarnation. I have asked myself this question so many times - why would I ever ask to be reincarnated in this tumultuous lifetime? I have been stuck by lightning and almost died, endured a life-ending brain aneurysm and other physical challenges, as well as almost losing my husband, John, to COVID-19.

The Angels have said that these extraordinary events have prepared all of us for meeting any challenges that will come up in the future. We each are to be beacons of light and love for all those around us. The stronger we are, the stronger our families and friends will be. It is a matter of exchanging energy from one person to another. What if we could gift freedom, bravery and joy to others? How dynamic would that be! Be the light! Be the example! You are extraordinary! Doing extraordinary work just by being here! The Angels salute you and send you deep love!

Namaste (the Divine in me, celebrates the Divine in you) to you and yours!

BE FEARLESS
IN THE PURSUIT OF
WHAT SETS YOUR SOUL
ON FIRE

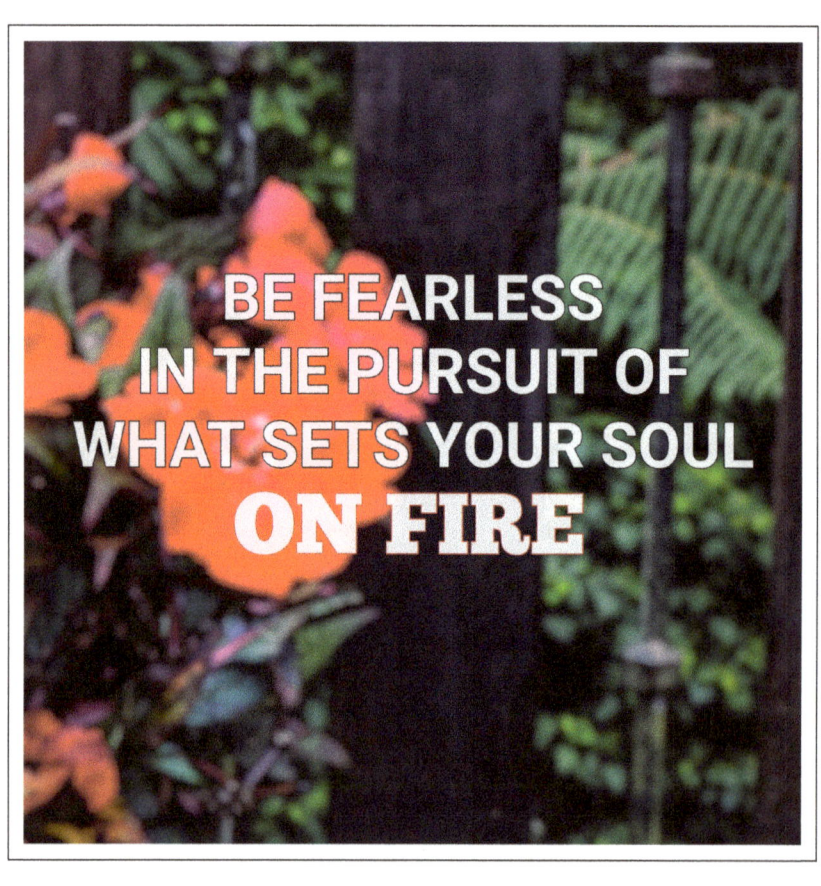

Blog #6

Being Human is No Cake Walk!

From the Angels:
"Why do you think you volunteered to be born into this chaotic time?
(See Angelic Blog #5).

This is a tough Soul assignment to be in a physical body with all of its challenges and a need to be energetic, healthy, wise and loving. Life just doesn't give you a golden wand and off you go to sprinkle positive fairy dust. I know Sue is finding this assignment of being human exceedingly difficult right now. Ill loved ones, financial challenges, a new business to get off the ground - just like so many of you. She knows it is for the better but still just wants peace and serenity - the way it was before! But that's not the assignment for 2020. The mission for 2020 and beyond is to bring peace and love to all of the beings on the planet - a pretty big deal! So, how do you do that in your own way? Here are a few suggestions that might help from us, your Angelic friends:

- <u>Smile</u>—the energy from your smile uplifts others and yourself. It brings joy to the planet and is infectious.
- <u>Breathe</u> - your breath is the breath of God. Keep it going in and out of your body. A strong body allows Universal energy to permeate every cell.

- <u>Pray</u>—prayer is a conversation with God and this extraordinary Angelic realm. We are here for you and want to help you through these massive changes.

- <u>Believe</u> - these changes and challenges are for humanity's betterment toward an all-loving earth. All things that are not of the loving Light will be eliminated. It just takes time.

- <u>Offer Gratitude</u> - every time you are grateful for what you have, what you are doing that you love, or for those you love, this magnetic vibration comes back to you in greater quantity.

- <u>Discover a new life:</u> Find the positive in every situation. You will always learn something new about how strong you really are and what you can accomplish.

We wish you a safe journey and until next time,
Be safe! Be healthy! And, know that you are loved beyond measure!"

With love and light,

Your Angelic Friends

Freedom
is a State
of
Mind

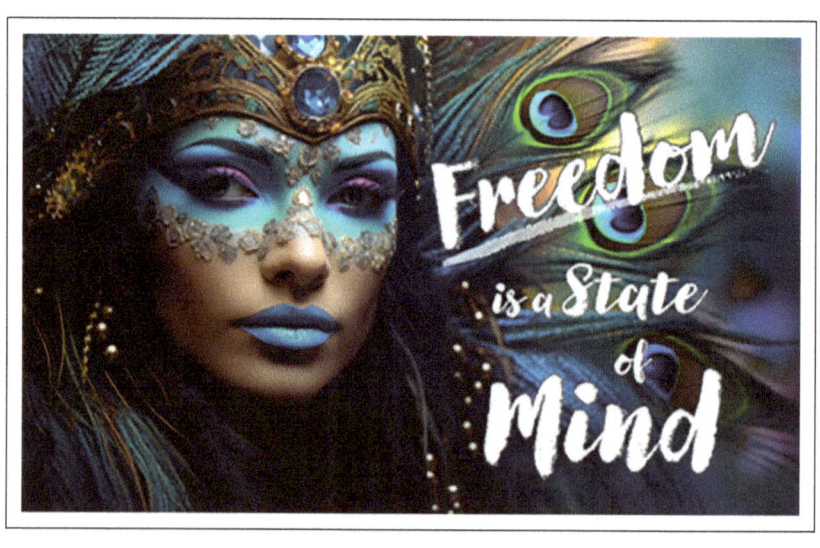

Blog #7

2020

WE Are Becoming a DIY Society! More Freedom, More Personal Power!

What is a DIY Society? It is a society of people who are "Do It Yourself" and want their personal freedom at the forefront of their lives. We are learning more about ourselves and what we are capable of every day, especially during challenging times like COVID-19. If you read Angelic Message #1, you will see that the information I relay to you is with the guidance of the Angelic realm that lives with us every minute of every day. I do not know who these extraordinary beings are because so many different ones have come to me over the years, in visual and auditory connection. I so hope you enjoy their Words of Wisdom.

DIY is all about these revelations:

- "You are extraordinary and capable of so much more than you know."
- "No one else can define your gifts and talents - only you."
- "Live from the inside out - from your heart vs. your brain. The heart has a brain of its own."
- "ALWAYS love yourself first. You will then feel '*I can vs. I can't.*'"

- "You can love others as you love yourself."
- "Follow no one else except your own intuition/heart."
- "Just as you are learning to work from home, cutting your own and your family's hair, finding REAL time for connecting to those you love - you will learn to rely more on your own guidance because you will have the time to reflect."
- "An empowered society is one who does not rely on others to create their future."
- *"Be safe, be well. Know that you are loved beyond measure!"*

From Sue:

- We will learn to follow business and personal paths that most excite and challenge us vs. just doing the same thing every day. Our passion for our lives ignites the passion in others. Our reliance on outside countries to build economic freedom has jailed us to the dictates of others. *We are independent, free-thinking Americans who can create exactly the lives we want to live. This is a time for re-inventing who we are.*
- *You are extraordinary! Follow your dreams! Do not allow challenges like COVID-19 to cause you to feel that your life today is over—it is, but in a good way. New dreams are emerging, and new opportunities are coming!*

Be there for your NEW DIY spirit!

All the strength
you need
is within you.
Your inner world
is YOUR domain.
Gordana Biernat
mypowertalk.com

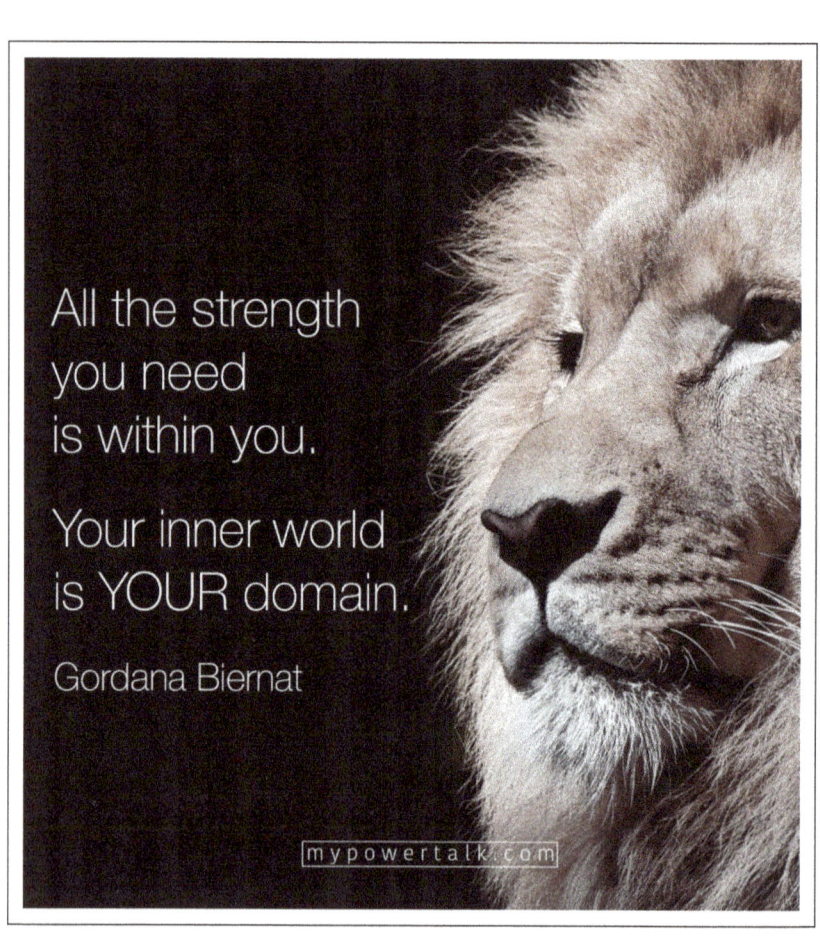

Blog #8

Creating Greater Personal Freedom!

From the Angels:
"You are extraordinary! What has 2020 taught you? What have you learned? We see so many humans wondering what has happened. Why so much change, so much sadness, so much loss? This, Beloveds, is a global reset. This is all about you, as human beings, living from the inside out - from the heart instead of the head. Love each other and all beings regardless of skin color, beliefs, or origin. You are ALL extraordinary beings because you volunteered to be here at this time of enormous change and personal chaos. We thank you deeply!

Now, what do you do with the wisdom that you have gleaned during 2020? Do you appreciate more? Do you have greater gratitude for what is present in your life? And love more than before because you have seen how precious human life can be. We don't need you on 'our side' yet. We need you on the earth plane. What we are asking of you in 2021 and beyond is to be completely independent in your thinking and actions. Live from your deep intuition when it comes to the decisions you make in your life:

- Vaccines: yes or no
- Health decisions: yes or no

- Future work/career choices
- Politics
- Living a simpler, more fulfilling life

This is all about letting go of FEAR of the future and letting bravery take its place. You are extraordinary! Be safe! Be well! And know that you are loved beyond measure!"

From Sue:
This new year of 2021 will challenge us all to listen to the heart and its guidance. Not to let the media, the political rhetoric and the fear of the future drive our decisions. As I have said before, with the Angels nodding 'yes', being human during this historical time is not for sissies!

Sending each of you love and gratitude for who you are and for being here at this time!

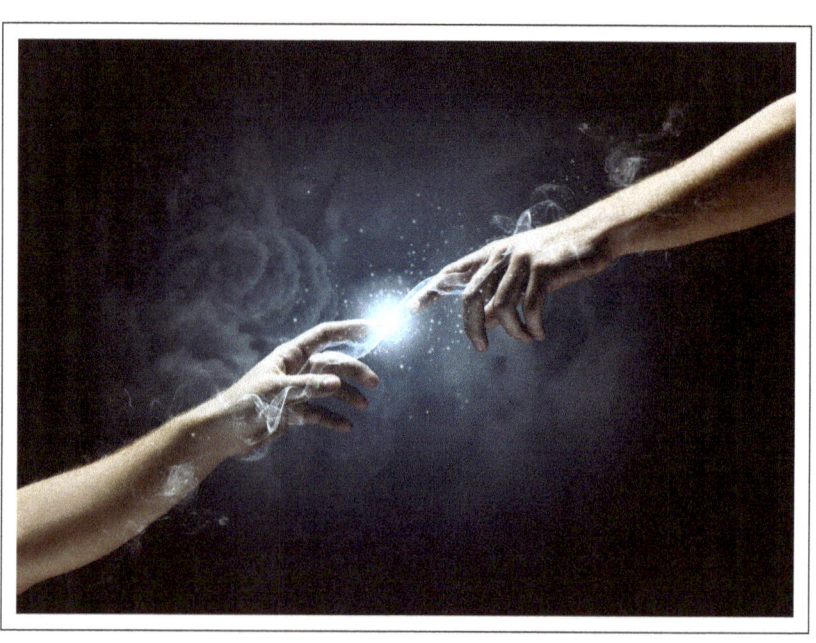

Blog #9

Your God Connection

From Sue and the Angels:
"You are extraordinary! You (your soul) volunteered to be born into this earthly life and be here to assist in these enormous global changes. We are sure you are asking - how? By just being you - the passionate and loving version of yourself that is being called upon to take your born-given gifts and talents and share them with the world. Again, you may ask - how? By experimenting with all of the things that give you joy. Do you like to paint, write, dance, teach, heal, lead, build businesses, speak, love animals, love sports, cook - what gifts can you share? What did you love to do as a child? What books, magazines and blogs do you read? What shows, movies and videos do you like to view? What lights you up? What excites those around you? Write them down. Study them. You will see a pattern of your passions. Then, act on them and share them.

What does any of the above have to do with God? How are you connected to God when you follow your passions? That is why we, as Angel messengers, have come into your lives through these blogs from Sue. She is a bridge from the physical to the non-physical worlds. You are connected to God and the Angelic realm because you bring healing, peace, and joy to the world around you when you share your gifts and talents. The "veil" between the physical and nonphysical worlds has become thinner and connection can now become so much more real. You are *always* connected; just now, it will seem more real. Try it! *Feel* what it is like to talk to us, connect with us, trust us. Your intuition will help you do this. Trust yourself!

We wish you a safe journey, and until next time, Be safe! Be healthy! And know that you are loved beyond measure!"

With love and gratitude for your journey, Your Angelic Friends

part three

DANCING WITH THE DIVINE

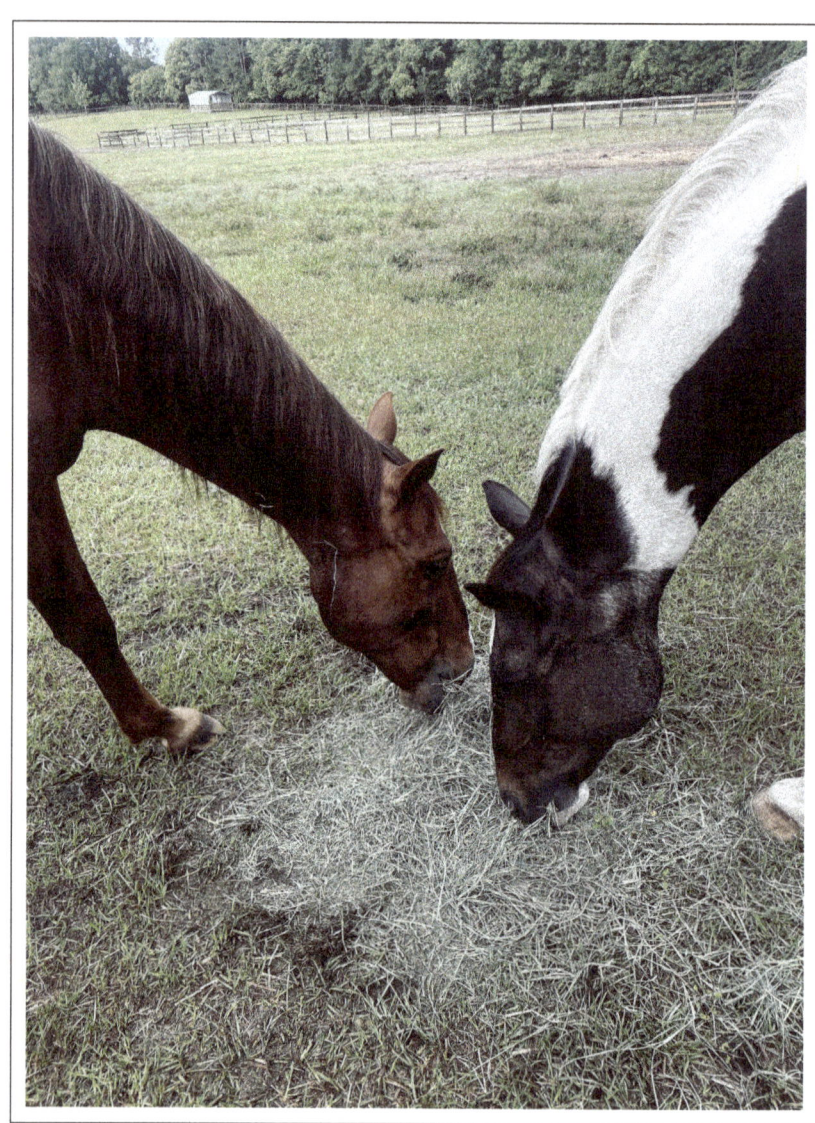

part three

DANCING WITH THE DIVINE

Now that you've had a chance to connect with the Divine through my encounters, I want you to know that your Dancing with the Divine comes through the passion you feel for life and through sharing your gifts and talents with the world. You are an extension of Source energy, and you volunteered for this lifetime to live on the edge of life's experiences and to represent a Dance with the Divine.

What are your gifts and talents? What do you love to do most? What books do you read? What movies do you see, and what podcasts do you listen to? These avenues will tell you what you are here to do if you don't already know. Mother Nature is the catalyst for opening up our hearts and helping us discover what our divinity wants us to do for the world. For me, it is with my horses, The Fabulous Five. Every time I am with them, I must be my best self. To be calm and grounded. To be kind and generous in my interactions with them. To be aware of their world and how they relate with each other. The lead mare, Skye, keeps everyone in line, especially the "boys" (geldings). They are not to be selfish at the water trough or pushy in the run-in during severe weather. They are to share their hay on the ground with those horses they feel comfortable with. So, as I watch them, I ask myself what lessons can I learn? Have I been the kindest and most compassionate I could be?

Have I shared my gifts and talents – my "hay"? What fear can I release so that I can offer my gifts to the world? All of these questions are what I ask myself daily. So, let's look at the how-to's of finding your passion in the Divine Dance that the Angels share with us:

The "How To's" of the Divine Dance:

- You take the "lead" in this dance by being in touch with your "inner being" every time you have a question about life. Your "inner being" (your soul) is your intuition. Your intuitive hits from your soul are your guideposts along the way.

- !0% of your inner being is here in this earthly realm, and 90% is on the "other side." The "other side" is where all of your soul came from and where 90% of it now resides, waiting to connect with you anytime you want its love and counsel.

- Your 10% is the creator of your life and the 90% is your wisdom and guidance. Soul 90% gathers insight and knowledge for you. Your job is to tap into its connection.

- How to "tap into"? Feel where the messages are experienced in your body? The stomach: leading you to greater personal power. The heart: loving the concept or path you are deliberating. The brain (the worry wart): allow it to rest and feel the energy of the heart, which has a brain of its own. Forget the worry about the future or the "what ifs." The thyroid and endocrine system: speak up. Put your "big girl panties" on! You are important to this world. Your feelings and thoughts matter!

- Every day, spend time in nature. Your breath is the breath of God. Breathe in, breathe out. Smell the flowers, feel the rain, snow or sunshine on your face. Love your animals—pause for a moment and hold them and feel their hearts beat. They are emitting the energy of love to you. They know why they are here—to help you connect with ALL of yourself. All lives matter—all four-legged and two-legged lives are God's children.

- Say "yes" to opportunities that come your way, even if you feel that you are not ready for them. You will learn as you go.

Am I going as far as I can with all that I've got?

Are you? Are you Dancing with the Divine as your unique, glorious self? Are you going as far as you can with all that you've got? I know you are. You are EXTRAORDINARY! As I have been editing this book, I realized that both the lightning accident and the brain aneurysm were invasions of light entering my body to help me recognize that I have a contract with the Universe. My job is to fulfill my purpose of sharing the awareness that Angels and the Divine are real; your purpose and passion to elevate the energy of our world are real.

Your soul was chosen over hundreds of thousands of souls to reincarnate into this world *at this time.* Now, what are you going to do with this gift of life?

I challenge you to "Light Your Life on Fire!"

IN GRATITUDE

In Gratitude

As I began to recount all of the extraordinary people who have helped me and given me guidance over the last ten years about honoring my Angelic experiences, I saw my mother saying, "Sue, you can do this. Take your love of the Universe and Mother Nature, and spread that love to others." She passed at age 96, a lifelong lover of horses, golf and the great outdoors.

I also deeply thank my husband, John, for giving me much-needed loving encouragement and time and space to write and think when I could have been spending time with him. Thank you, Darling!

And to my two adult children, Chris and Cathy, for your encouragement over the years to not only be your mother but a good friend who had talents to share with the world—I love you more than life itself. Thank you from the bottom of my heart for being the extraordinary people you are.

To my life coach and mentor, Lisa Howell (www.healthierwayscoaching.com) – you are an extraordinary healer and I am so blessed to have you and your healing energy in my life. Thank you for being YOU!

To my friends, Charlie and Maryam, who guided me with all of their gifted IT support – thank you!

To the encouragement of my horse-related friends who cheered me on as I wove my stories into the Angelic and equine experience of a lifetime.

And, to all of my friends and family members, I love you and thank you for being your unique selves and in my life.

Images

- Page 2: Courtesy of Shutterstock
- Page 6: Courtesy of Shutterstock
- Page 12: Courtesy of LDR Media
- Page 18: Courtesy of LDR Media
- Page 20: Courtesy of Marcello Mancinelli Photography, "Age of Innocence"
- Page 24: Courtesy of Erin Hanson, poet, and horse tricks 101
- Page 28: Courtesy of LDR Media
- Page 30: Courtesy of Shutterstock
- Page 34: Courtesy of LDR Media
- Page 38: Courtesy of LDR Media
- Page 42: Courtesy of LDR Media
- Page 46: Courtesy of Gordana Biernat: mypowertalk.com
- Page 50: Courtesy of Shutterstock: Michaelangelo's God's Touch
- Page 54: Courtesy of LDR Media: Bandit and Nic sharing their "hay": passion for living

www.ingramcontent.com/pod-product-compliance
Lightning Source LLC
Chambersburg PA
CBHW051603010526
44118CB00023B/2797